How To Stop Hair Loss In Women

by Sabrina R Perkins

No more suffering in Silence

Contents

Olive Oil

Castor Oil

Lavender Oil

Sweet Almond Oil

Scalp Massages

Consult a professional

Try new and promising treatments

More Resources

Black Women & Hair Loss

Seriously Natural Blog

Natural Hair For Beginners Blog

Dedication

I am dedicating this book to children, Matt, Megan & Taylen. While all three contribute to my growing numbers of gray hair, I love them all with every fiber of my being. Thank you to all three for keeping me creative.

Introduction

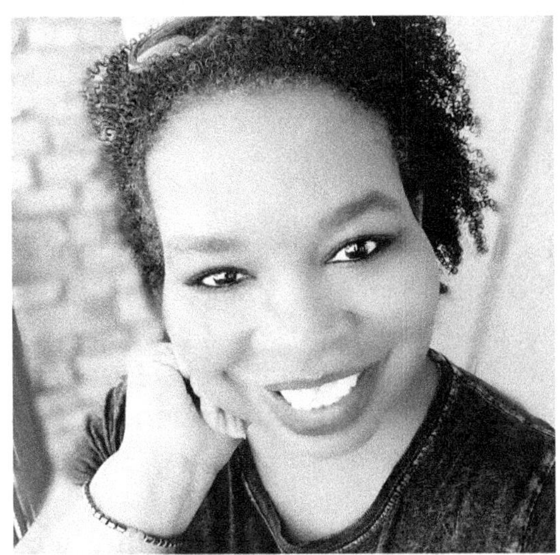

Welcome to *How To Stop Hair Loss In Women* by me, Sabrina R Perkins, a natural hair and beauty blogger with two successful blogs, seriouslynatural.org and naturalhairforbeginners.com

This Book is a quick and easy tool for not just stopping hair loss, but to understand what it is and how to defeat it successfully. All too often women are being silent on hair loss and it's time to open our mouths for help and gain solid and accurate knowledge to regaining our healthy strands and beautiful hair.

I KNOW this Book with be a great asset to ridding yourself of hair loss and regaining the confidence and beautiful hair you deserve!

Sabrina

Chapter 1: What Is Hair Loss?

Believed to affect mostly men but can and does affect women, hair loss is defined as:

> "Hair loss is the thinning of hair on the scalp. The medical term for hair loss is alopecia. Alopecia can be temporary or permanent. The most common form of hair loss occurs gradually and is referred to as "androgenetic alopecia," meaning that a combination of hormones (androgens are male hormones) and heredity (genetics) is needed to develop the condition. Other types of hair loss include alopecia areata (patches of baldness that usually grow back), telogen effluvium (rapid shedding after childbirth, fever, or sudden weight loss); and traction alopecia (thinning from tight braids or ponytails)." [1]

---

[1] (n.d.). Definition of Hair loss - MedicineNet. Retrieved March 20, 2018, from https://www.medicinenet.com/script/main/art.asp?articlek ey=53390

Chapter 2: Why Do Women Suffer From Hair Loss?

Most women will suffer from some sort of hair loss within their lifetime. From hair thinning to hair fall, women have often thought this was more of a problem for men and didn't really concern them. Sorry, but many of the very products you've been using over the years have slowly been depleting the hair of its protein and oils that it desperately needs to grow strong and fight off damage, dryness and hair loss. From hair coloring to hair straightening, we've been chipping away at the hair's cuticle and if we are not rebuilding those strands, we are leaving them helpless and ripe for damage.

Even if you are taking medications for certain illnesses that are necessary, taking out the time to speak with a physician is advised because they can offer more natural approaches that have will have a much less negative impact on your hair growth. If you are suffering from above average hair loss and want to take back control of the situation, there are several options to fix the problem. First, let's learn more about why women even suffer from hair loss i the first place.

In 2016, a consumer survey conducted by Keranique® – the Women's Hair Growth Experts™ sheds light on the alarming numbers of American women who have experienced hair loss. According to the survey:

- Nearly 40% of U.S. women 18+ have noticed signs of hair loss or thinning

- Over 50% of US women 58 or older have experienced it
- That number jumps to over 60% for women age 65+
- These signs include: a widening part, hair being thinner than it used to be, significant signs of overall hair loss, and seeing through to the scalp where they couldn't before especially in the temples or at the crown of the head.

Who is at risk?

Research indicates women in one or more of these 3 categories are more susceptible to hair loss and thinning:

- Women are 97% more likely (almost twice as likely) to experience signs of hair loss if they have a relative with hair loss compared to those who don't, and 61% of women who have relatives with hair loss are experiencing symptoms of hair loss.
- Women who have had chemical treatments are 71% more likely to experience hair loss than those who have not, and over half (58%) of women who have had chemical treatments are experiencing signs of hair loss.
- Women who have been ill or taking medicine are 81% more likely to suffer from hair loss and thinning than

those who have not, and over half (58%) of women who have been ill or taking medicine are experiencing signs of hair loss.

- And many could be at risk for future issues. 62% of women have noticed changes to their hair just in the past year. [2]

Why so many? Well, a few factors include unhealthy hair habits, stress, and women not seeking help are all reasons for such devastating numbers. Ways to beat this are enlisting good hair habits with healthy hair education, living a healthier lifestyle, and seeking professional help from a physician, dermatologist or a Trichologist are all excellent ways to combat the problem.

---

[2] (2016, August 1). More Than 46 Million American Women Across the US Affected By .... Retrieved March 20, 2018, from https://www.prnewswire.com/news-releases/more-than-46-million-american-women-across-the-us-affected-by-hair-loss-more-at-risk-300306419.html

What are the reasons black women suffer MORE from hair loss?

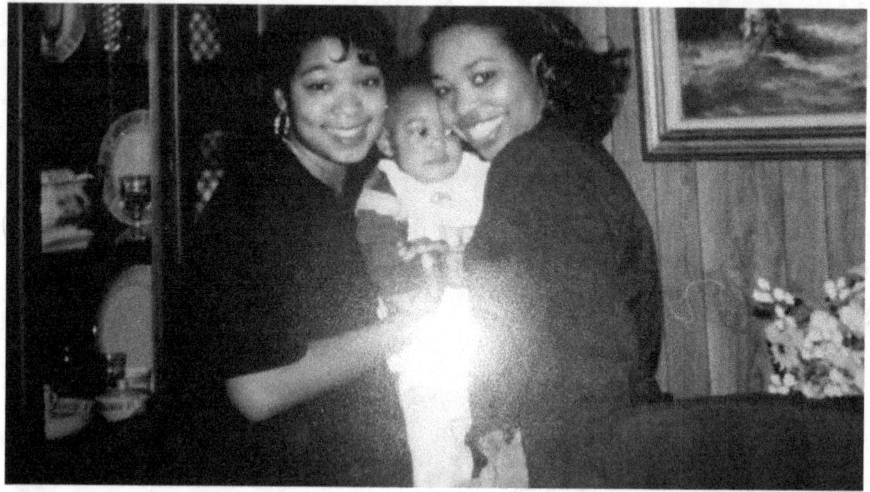

Hair loss is a serious subject that far too many women face. It would be neglectful of me as a black woman to NOT discuss a recent study presented at the American Academy of Dermatology Annual Meeting that black women are more prone to hair loss. Another study in 2016 at the American Academy of Dermatology's 74th Annual Meeting in Washington showed that black women are more prone to hair loss. They also found that even though we are prone to hair loss, we are less likely to seek professional help.

Learn more about Black Women & Hair Loss in my new book on kindle and in paperback,
Black Women & Hair Loss: How to Stop Losing Our Hair & Gain Maximum Hair Growth

Chapter 3: What May Be Causing Your Hair Loss

We've discussed top reasons but there may be more reasons as to why some women are suffering from hair loss, hair thinning or even just damaged hair.

Anemia

Anemia, simply put is a low iron intake. Not getting enough iron in your diet and couple that with a heavy menstruation flow can cause this problem and this may result in inadequate folic acid.

According to research at WebMD[3] on Anemia, the body begins to produce lower levels of hemoglobin, and that can eventually result in some women suffering from hair loss due to a lack of oxygen to the hair follicles. This makes the hair weaker and easier to break. If the condition persists, hair loss will become more pronounced.

---

[3] (2016, June 26). Anemia Causes, Types, Symptoms, Diet, and Treatment - WebMD. Retrieved March 29, 2018, from https://www.webmd.com/a-to-z-guides/understanding-anemia-basics

Damaging Hair Practices

For many women, they don't even realize that they are causing their own hair loss because of poor hair practices like over processing hair with chemicals from color, hair straightening or perms. Using too much heat, especially without using heat protectants can also weaken the hair and cause breakage or hair loss.   Now that weaker and brittle hair is exposed to products with harsh chemicals that further weaker and damage the hair.

Effects Of Menopause

One of the things you cannot avoid when it comes to common concern for women and hair loss is how menopause may affect your body.
According to Healthline,

> "Research suggests that hair loss during menopause is the result of a hormonal imbalance. Specifically, it's related to a lowered production of estrogen and progesterone. These hormones help hair grow faster and stay on the head for longer periods of time. When the levels of estrogen and progesterone drop, hair grows more slowly and becomes much thinner.

A decrease in these hormones also triggers an
increase in the production of androgens, or a
group of male hormones. Androgens shrink
hair follicles, resulting in hair loss on the head.
In some cases, however, these hormones can
cause more hair to grow on the face. This is
why some menopausal women develop facial
"peach fuzz" and small sprouts of hair on the
chin."[4]

Powerful Medications

Unfortunately, some of the very medicines we need to stay
alive or even just stay healthy can cause subtle to severe hair
loss when taking them. Discussing your medications that may
cause side effects of hair loss with your doctor is the best way
to deal with this issue as there may be alternative meds to try.
You are your own advocate so talk to your PCP and see what,
if anything, can be done if you sense your hair loss may be
due to your meds. Make sure to check out the side effects of
your meds as a little research will yield what may be causing
this problem.

---

[4] (2016, January 19). Hair Loss and Menopause - Healthline.
Retrieved March 29, 2018, from
https://www.healthline.com/health/menopause/hair-loss

Extreme Weight Loss

Crash diets, long fasting or just not eating is one of the worst ways to lose weight but they also can cause damage to your body, especially when it comes to your hair. Losing too much weight suddenly may seem attractive but it may be at the expense of your hair. Crash diets deprive the body of those proteins, and that can weaken your strands. When you try to lose too much weight too fast, you are depriving your body of vital nutrients, all of which have a negative impact on hair growth.

The Aging Process

Hair loss can be devastating at any age, but there are ways to prevent it. As we get older, the hair strands weaken causing an increase in breakage and thinning. Usually a result of hormonal changes in the body, the levels of estrogen (which promotes thick hair) we produce begins to decline as we get older. Women also begin to process nutrients less efficiently as we grow older, so diet is crucial to stay healthy and that directly relates to our hair.

Chapter 4: How To Stop Hair Loss & Encourage Hair Growth

We've discussed what many women who suffer from hair loss can attribute to the problem, but how can we stop it? How to stop hair loss is one of the biggest concerns for any woman suffering from it. You want answers and solutions that are quick and easy but like anything else in life, it can take time. We do have proven solutions that will reverse the damage and allow your hair to thrive.

Ginger

Many of us know how amazing ginger is and use it often in the kitchen but did you know it was also great for our hair? This wonderful natural root has lots of uses in the culinary world, but it also helps relieve minor stomach ailments. This root is part of the Zingiberaceae family, along with cardamom and turmeric. It is commonly produced in India, Jamaica, Fiji, Indonesia, and Australia. From face masks to moisturizers, people have been applying this potent spice to their skin and hair for centuries.

One of the best things about ginger when it comes to beauty is its effect on hair. If you are one of the many people currently suffering from hair loss it may be a useful thing to try. Whether you have long, straight locks or gorgeous curls like 4a hair, ginger has a lot to offer. Ginger has a range of benefits for the scalp, roots and ends of hair, from stopping thinning to increasing blood flow and giving the hair much needed minerals. Check out this great hair recipe for encouraging hair growth.

Ginger + Coconut Oil Hair Growth Mask

<u>Ingredients:</u>
1 Tbsp. finely grated Ginger
2 Tbsp. warmed slightly Coconut oil or Sesame oil
Cheesecloth or Muslin cloth

<u>Method:</u>
Blend the ginger into a fine paste before squeezing out the juice the cheesecloth or muslin cloth. Set the ginger juice to the side as you will be using it later. Combine the squeezed-out ginger and coconut oil together until well mixed. Add the ginger juice and still well.

<u>How to use:</u>
Use before washing hair by massaging the mixture into your scalp well. Cover with a plastic cap and leave in for at least one hour. Wash out with shampoo and style as usual.

Hair Tea Rinses

Tea rinses are gaining ground in the natural hair movement. Hibiscus tea benefits are well documented but when it comes to hair teas, there are several types of teas that are beneficial. First off, these aren't really teas at all but instead, infusions of leaves, bark, roots, fruits or flowers of nearly any edible, non-tea plant. These infusions of herbs can do wonders for our bodies and they most certainly help to achieve beautiful hair. You don't even have to harness their goodness just by drinking. Let's delve into the world of hair teas.

A hair tea or hair tea rinse is simply brewing a type of tea, allowing it to steep and cool prior to pouring it over your hair and scalp. Massaging your scalp with the hair tea is next and this all happens after hair has been washed. Teas are great for not only stimulating hair growth but also for coloring hair, aiding some scalp issues and even hair thickening. Black tea is a favorite for hair growth as it is high in caffeine and a simple tea rinse after washing your hair is a wonderful way to regularly fight hair loss.

Natural Oils

Natural oils, both essential and carrier hold a host of components that fight hair loss and even stimulate hair growth. Here is a list of some of the best natural oils for fighting hair loss.

Coconut Oil

Coconut oil contains Lauric acid which fights off various bacteria and fungi that can be found on the irritated scalps. Infections of the scalp can cause a significant amount of hair fall, as the follicles shed as they become swollen and irritated. Coconut oil is also known as the only oil that can fully penetrate the hair follicle, rebuilding it from the inside out and reducing the likelihood of unnecessary damage.

Olive Oil

Often used for cooking and salad dressings, olive oil is one of the most common household oils that can be found. Not only does it make a great vinaigrette, but it also contains an impressive amount of vitamin E and other monounsaturated fatty acids that promote hair growth and reduce hair fall. Of course, the more expensive and pure the olive oil is, the more vitamins and nutrient it will contain, so you may need to pay a pretty penny if you're looking for the top-notch results.

Castor Oil

Aside from causing an impressive "internal cleansing" ingredient, this oil also contains hair growth and regeneration properties. The oil's triglycerides of ricinoleic acid makes it anti-fungal, anti-bacterial and anti-inflammatory, which are all important components that are needed to both combat and prevent scalp infections, fungi and unhealthy bacteria. The restorative properties of castor oil strengthen the roots of the hair, therefore reducing shedding, while also causing new hairs to grow in quick, thick, and much healthier. Many women are finding the best way to regrow edges is by using Jamaican Black Castor Oil for scalp massages.

Lavender Oil

Lavender oil is stimulating, meaning that it increases circulation to the scalp. Not only does that encourage new hair growth, but it also provides much needed nutrients and oxygen to the roots of the hair, which makes the root stronger and reduces the amount of shedding. This oil also combats against nits and lice, which is something else that can lead to hair fall. Much like its counterparts, it also contains antibacterial properties that wards off infections, fungi and unwanted bacteria.

Sweet Almond Oil

Almond oil is known to be a natural "moisturizer" due to its softening properties. Containing Vitamins E and D, along a host of other minerals such as calcium and magnesium, makes almond oil one of the only oils that can prevent the hair from drying out and becoming brittle. Dry, brittle hair tends to break and fall out very easily.

Incorporating sweet almond oil into your regimen will not only provide your hair with some much-needed nutrition, but it will also ensure that the hair stays strong and grows in faster.

Scalp Massages

Aside from being incredibly relaxing, regular scalp massages (at least 3x a week) can help prevent hair loss as well as encourage healthy hair growth. Massaging the scalp promotes blood flow which provides the scalp with oxygen and other nutrients that are beneficial to maintaining healthy roots. This also encourages a healthy production of sebum-the natural oil produced by the scalp. Although our oil glands shrink gradually as we age, the oil can always be supplemented with other natural oils. Using oils such as castor, lavender, peppermint, or cayenne can heighten the effectiveness of the massage by stimulating the scalp and further increasing the amount of blood flow to the roots of the hair. All the oils mentioned above are excellent for scalp massages.

Consult a professional

Sometimes we need to bring in the big guns and that means consulting a Dermatologist, MD, Trichologist or professional hairstylist.   These professionals can see if your hair loss is attributed to a medical condition, medication or if medicines need to be prescribed to stop the hair loss and to aid in regrowing your hair. Our lifestyle, age, and health can directly affect our hair positively and negatively so consult the professional to ensure you are doing everything possible for healthy scalp and hair.

Try new and promising treatments

The beauty market continues to assist women in hair loss remedies even if they seem to be muted in comparison to other ailments like anti-aging. One such promising treatments creating waves is PRP, or Platelet Rich Plasma Therapy. This treatment requires no surgery, no drugs and no expensive or messy ointments. While this treatment is new the process of Platelet Rich Plasma is not.

According to ABC News:

> "PRP starts by drawing blood from the patient. The blood then goes into a machine that separates out the platelets filled with growth factors. Those growth factor-filled platelets are then injected into the scalp to stimulate new-hair growth, decrease hair loss and make the hair grow thicker. Producing platelet rich plasma is approved by the Food and Drug Administration (FDA). The PRP procedure is not yet approved but there is a clinical trial underway now."[5]

---

[5] (2016, April 25). New Treatment Offers Hope for Women With Hair Loss - ABC News. Retrieved March 29, 2018, from http://abcnews.go.com/Health/treatment-offers-hope-women-hair-loss/story?id=38648107

Women in the study right now are seeing vast improvements and this was even discussed extensively on Good Morning America a few days ago. The treatments cost around $400 per session and the preliminary results look good but right not they are still just in the clinical trials. We can expect doctors to increase those prices enormously if all goes well with the trials.

More Resources

<u>Black Women & Hair Loss</u> How To Stop Losing Our Hair & Gain Massive Hair Growth

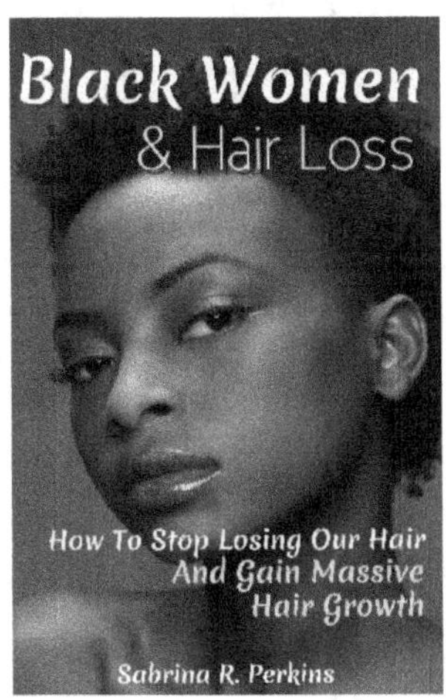

Black Women & Hair Loss is a new eBook by me, Sabrina R. Perkins where we are delving into the specifics of black hair and hair loss because this is a problem that far too many black women are facing.

This eBook is a quick and easy tool for not just stopping hair loss for Black women, but to understand what it is and how to defeat it successfully. All too often Black women are being silent on hair loss and it's time to open our mouths for help and gain solid and accurate knowledge to regaining our healthy strands and beautiful hair.

Thinning edges, resorting to weaves and wigs for length or severe breakage must be our reality. Learn how to win against hair loss with this Book.

Seriously Natural Blog

Seriously Natural is about Natural hair, beauty and style. From the basics to not so known tidbits; Seriously Natural brings all women the necessities to feel as lovely as they should with proper knowledge, tips and secrets that the experts know! Sharing information on very serious issues surrounding natural hair. I've also sprinkled extras in creativity, news, as well as health issues affecting the Black/African American community.

Natural Hair For Beginners Blog

Natural Hair For Beginners is for women of color who want to go natural but need solid tips to make their journey beautiful and positive. This is where you will get step by step instructions on how to go natural, what you use, when to use it and to ensure you are creating a positive space for your journey.

Thank You!

Thank you for your purchase!!! I would love for you to leave a review about this Book here: **How To Stop Hair Loss In Women Book**

Sabrina

Here's a sneak peek on my next book that out in April 2018.
21 Natural Hair Growth Stimulators.

Hair is an extension of our personality, our style, our being a woman. It can make a statement. It can become a shield. It can open the eyes of ridicule as easily as it can close the minds of disgust. It's more than protein strands and for many women it is about having a lot of it.

Therefore, I decided to create this book on the several natural methods that nature has to offer for growing it strong, long, and thick. I have tried a few of these myself with much success as well as others and with my 6+ years of researching, blogging, and freelance writing about hair and hair's health; I have found proven methods to do so.

I have listed the natural ingredients for optimal hair growth and a few recipes for the DIY lovers to tinker with for not only healthy hair but beautiful hair and skin to be fully proud of!

Chapter 1: Alfalfa Sprouts

More than that funny looking dude from the Lil Rascals, Alfalfa sprouts are not just for salads anymore! I tend to eat more bean sprouts in my Pho, but Alfalfa sprouts are where it's at! Alfalfa or Medicago sativa is a perennial, leguminous plant a part of the pea family and is a rapidly growing plant. They are easy to cultivate, are a deliciously crunchy and nutty tasting vegetable, and have a countless number of health-enhancing benefits.

Alfalfa sprouts are rich in vitamins A, B1, B6, C, E, and K.
They have calcium, carotene, iron, potassium, zinc and are an
excellent source of dietary fiber. They also contain protein
and for every serving of alfalfa sprouts provides 1 gram of
plant-based protein and because they can be eaten raw they
are great for people on vegan and raw diets.

Alfalfa Sprouts for Hair Growth
Alfalfa sprouts are excellent for combatting hair loss because
of the calcium, potassium magnesium, and folic acid.
Vitamins B1 and B6 both are important for the health of the
hair and vitamin C aids in improving scalp circulation which
brings the nutrients to the hair roots along with vitamin E that
increases the oxygen intake to the hair follicles. The full hair
growing ability of alfalfa sprouts are heightened when used in
conjunction with carrot and/or lettuce juice.

The best way to gain the benefits of Alfalfa Sprouts for your
hair is by eating them. You can add them to salads, soups and
sandwiches or simply add them to a favorite smoothie.
Another effortless way is to tap into this hair growing nutrient
is through juicing.

Alfalfa + Carrot Hair Growth Juice

What you need:
1 cup Alfalfa Sprouts
4-5 carrots
A few parsley leaves (optional)
Juicer

Method:
Place sprouts, carrots, and parsley in juicer. Mix and drink up
to 3 times a week for an increase in hair growth.

Chapter 2: Biotin

More than the word you hear about on every hair blog and vlog, Vitamin H, better known as Biotin, is a B complex vitamin that helps the body convert food into energy. A Biotin deficiency is rare as most people get their required amounts through healthy eating. Biotin can be naturally found in cauliflower, carrots, bananas, soy flower, liver, salmon, wheat germ and yeast just to name a few.

Biotin is a hugely popular supplement as many believe it to be excellent at increase hair and nail growth. Biotin can be found in conjunction with other vitamins for hair and nail vitamins or by itself.

Biotin For Hair Growth
There has not be extensive research on the effects of biotin on hair and nails despite the many claims to it positively increasing growth, strength for hair and nails. I have taken it while in hair vitamins and have seen an increase in nail strength and length and did see some hair growth.

Erica Douglas, fondly known as Sister Scientist, is a formulating cosmetic chemist with a degree in Chemical Engineering from Stanford University. She shares her thoughts on Biotin over at

I believe that biotin is most effective for the purposes of strengthening hair when used internally. Follicles of the hair are linked to blood vessels that absorb nutrients from the body. It's these nutrients that help to determine the hair's thickness and strength during the Anagen
phase of hair development.

Biotin Hair Supplements
The best way to get enough biotin in to help with hair is a supplement. It is a highly popular vitamin for hair, skin and nails and can be taken as a supplement alone, or in a multivitamin most often labeled as a hair, skin or nail vitamin. How much to take? Well, according to dermatologist Dr. Richard Scher, daily recommended dosage of biotin is 2.5 mg (or 2,500 mcg) but there has been no research on whether that is the right intake for optimal results from Biotin.

Chapter 3: Black Seed Oil

More than those annoying black seed found in our favorite summer treat watermelon, Black seed oil, also known as Black Coriander Oil or Black Cumin Seed oil, comes from seeds of the Nigella Sativa plant native to Asia. Part of the buttercup family, the plant has small, black, crescent shaped seeds and the use of these seeds date back to the times of King Tut in Ancient Egypt. Black seed oil is an essential oil and for naturalists it is often called the "cure for everything except death."

Black seed oil is an antioxidant, anti-bacterial, anti-inflammatory oil that fights infections and strengthens the human immune system. It has traditionally been used for digestive and gastrointestinal problems, headaches, colds, nasal congestion, allergies, and even hair and skin ailment.

Black Seed Oil For Hair Growth
 This is a great oil for overall improving hair health and fighting hair loss. It is often used in some cultures for fighting hair loss along with softening strands. While a great oil for hair because of its antioxidant and anti-bacterial properties, this oil is also loved for its ability to prevent premature graying. Simply applying the oil to hair and massaging aids in that plight.

Black Seed Oil Hair Treatment
What you need:
2 tbsp black seed oil

Method:
Pour the black seed oil into your palms of your hands and rub
them together to warm the oil. Massage the oil into your scalp
while focusing on the areas that are losing hair or need some
help with growth like edges. Once your scalp is covered in
the oil, work the oil through your hair from the roots to tips
and leave the oil in for about 30 minutes to an hour covered
with a plastic cap. Wash and style as usual.

www.ingramcontent.com/pod-product-compliance
Lightning Source LLC
Chambersburg PA
CBHW051928250726

48659CB00002B/903